Natalie Moore was born and raised in Halifax, West Yorkshire. The eldest of four, she has two sisters and one brother. She resides in her hometown where she enjoys walking and a regular iced-coffee!

I dedicate this book to all CFS/ME sufferers and to those struggling with their mental health.

Natalie Moore

THE IMPORTANCE OF REST

AUSTIN MACAULEY PUBLISHERS®

LONDON * CAMBRIDGE * NEW YORK * SHARJAH

A CIP catalogue record for this title is available from the British Library.

ISBN 9781035859078 (Paperback)
ISBN 9781035859108 (ePub e-book)

www.austinmacauley.com

First Published 2024
Austin Macauley Publishers Ltd®
1 Canada Square
Canary Wharf
London
E14 5AA

Scripture Quotation

Thank you to my friends and family who have helped encourage, and inspire me whilst writing this book.

Table of Contents

"Come to me all who are weary and heavy laden and I will give you rest." (Matthew 11: 28) NASB

Introduction

I had a dream to write this book when I was aged 30. The idea would come to me often but I never felt ready to start writing it. However, when I turned 31, the desire became stronger and so I decided to give it a go!

We live in a culture that thrives on 'busyness'. There's so much pressure in the world to keep pushing and striving for success. But this is not the way God wants us to live! Jesus took time to rest and be with His Heavenly Father and He wants us to do the same.

The Bible is a love story. It's a story about how our loving God tries to redeem His people by sending His own son, Jesus Christ to the cross to pay for our sins. He wants to bring us back home to Him and live with Him in Heaven for eternity.

When I was diagnosed with chronic fatigue syndrome/ME in 2012, my whole life changed. What I thought was going to be an overnight fix turned out to be a hard 10-year battle – not only for my physical health but, also my mental health.

I want you to know that this book has come from a place of deep pain – mental, emotional and physical. But it has also led me to experience the abundant peace and joy that Christ died to give us!

I have also had the wonderful privilege of coming to know the unrelenting love of our Heavenly Father who loves us so deeply.

I pray that this book will draw you closer to Jesus and that you will experience His love in ways you could never imagine!

Many blessings,
Natalie

My Story

I was just aged 21 when I was diagnosed with chronic fatigue syndrome/ME. At the time, I was working as a youth work trainee at a church in Wimborne, Dorset. Before I was diagnosed, I was very driven. I was very much an overachiever and worked at every opportunity I had. I started working from a young age at just 14 years old. I also went to a grammar school where there was a lot of pressure to achieve exceptionally high grades. If I wasn't working, studying or volunteering, I was out partying a lot from a young age too.

I didn't know the meaning of rest! I thought I just had to keep going and going. Until my body couldn't handle it anymore.

Unfortunately, there is a lot of stigma surrounding chronic fatigue syndrome/ME still. I would get comments when I was initially diagnosed like, "Aren't you just a bit depressed?" Or "I get tired too." This was incredibly frustrating and I began to feel very alone. Especially as there wasn't much help out there for CFS/ME sufferers.

I'd had dreams that in my 20s I would be doing what most people were doing my age. Before I was a youth worker, I studied at a prestigious university. I absolutely loved my time there and wouldn't change any of it! But I had hoped I would get a high-flying job and travel the world once I graduated. But, the reality of living with CFS/ME soon hit home and I began to realise that my dreams weren't going to happen anytime soon.

As a result of this crushing reality, I sank into a severe depression. I would go through episodes of severe depression but, then I would have times where I seemed to be doing better. There were also times when I got referred to CFS/ME clinics and I had the help of online support groups. However, depression got the better of me in 2018 when I was admitted to a mental health hospital where I spent nearly two years.

I didn't see it coming! But I didn't realise how unwell I was. When I was in hospital, I started taking drugs and turning to alcohol to try and cope with what I was going through. I was also self-harming and having suicidal thoughts. But it wasn't until I took a massive overdose and nearly lost my life, that I realised something needed to change.

After surviving the huge overdose, I decided to meet with the local chaplain at the hospital. He was a lovely man and he prayed for me. I felt a weight off my shoulders when he did! But I was still struggling with guilt and shame over the things I had done in the past.

I started to feel depressed again but then I heard about a friend I'd met in the hospital who had taken his own life. It made me realise that I didn't want my life to end the same way. So, I started reading God's word out loud, praying, worshipping and seeking God.

Suddenly, I came to a new beginning! And things started to change. I got referred back to a well-known chronic fatigue specialist who has helped me immensely. She also recommended a dietitian to me as I'd been having ongoing digestive issues too. Plus, my mental health team have been amazingly supportive and I finally feel like things are moving forward positively for me now.

Since I've been doing a lot better and I'm in a much better place mentally and physically. Although I still have CFS/ME, it's not as severe as it once was and I am able to manage it as well as my mental health much better than before.

The aim of this book is to share with you the many lessons I have learned over the years about managing CFS/ME, depression and anxiety. But, also to teach the importance of rest and self-care. As I shared before, we live in a world full of pressure and worry. But God wants us to look after ourselves and when we do that, we can better love others too. After all, the second commandment is to love your neighbour as yourself! (Mark 12: 31).

I will also draw on bible stories about characters who have faced similar trials but, whose stories always end well. I hope this will be an encouragement to you!

What is CFS/ME?

Chronic Fatigue Syndrome (also known as Myalgic Encephalomyelitis) is a long-term health condition characterised by many different symptoms.

Some of these symptoms include:

- ➢ Extreme fatigue which doesn't improve with rest
- ➢ Malaise – generally feeling unwell
- ➢ Headaches or migraines
- ➢ Insomnia or oversleeping
- ➢ Problems with memory and/or concentration
- ➢ Sensitivity to light and noise
- ➢ Muscle or joint pain
- ➢ A sore throat
- ➢ Flu-like symptoms
- ➢ Nausea
- ➢ Heart palpitations

Some people also develop depression and anxiety as a result of living with chronic fatigue syndrome.

In my case, I caught the flu virus before I was diagnosed with CFS/ME. Statistics show that about 5% of CFS/ME sufferers make a full recovery. So, for many sufferers this becomes an illness they have to learn to live with and manage on a daily basis.

Living with CFS/ME

Due to the debilitating and fluctuating nature of CFS/ME, this can be an incredibly hard illness to live with. Here are some of the emotions I have experienced whilst, living with it.

Anger

"I don't want to go through this anymore!" is something I would often feel. Living with CFS/ME can be extremely painful not just physically but emotionally too. Sometimes when I was really struggling with CFS/ME and depression, I would just ask God to take me home to be with Him in Heaven so I wouldn't have to suffer anymore. But I had to learn that God has a purpose for me whilst I'm here on this earth and I cannot go home until that purpose has been fulfilled.

Frustration

Frustration has been one of the hardest emotions for me to deal with. Having always been a 'doer' before I was diagnosed with CFS/ME, I would really struggle with the limits this condition put on my life. As I had to be very disciplined in learning to rest, I would often feel annoyed as sometimes I just didn't want to rest! I wanted to do something.

I would often pray to God about my frustrations. This helped lift the weight of dealing with the emotion of frustration.

Loneliness

As a single person living with CFS/ME, I struggled a lot with loneliness. The ongoing stigma that surrounds chronic fatigue syndrome can add to feelings of loneliness and isolation too. The promise that Jesus is always with me has given me great comfort during these periods of loneliness and isolation. I will talk more later on how to manage loneliness but, one way is by talking to Jesus about it. He understands loneliness. He understood it when he hung on the cross for our sins and when he was deserted by his disciples. *"And surely I am with you always, to the very end of the age."* *(Matthew 28: 20)* NIV

Disappointment

"Though he slay me, yet will I hope in him." *(Job 13: 15)* NIV

We all go through seasons of disappointment. Living with chronic illness can provoke feelings of disappointment especially as life may not have turned out the way we had hoped. Disappointment can be painful! But the good news is God doesn't waste our disappointment. We can turn it over to Him and allow Him to bring something good from it.

Sadness

"Weeping may last through the night, but joy comes with the morning." (Psalm 30: 5) NLT. Seeing other people who were my age getting married and travelling the world was a great source of disappointment for me. I would often feel resentful that others could do the things that I wanted to do. Of course, I am still hoping for these things in the future but, during my time of not being able to do any of these things, I would often feel a great deal of sadness.

Maybe you too are struggling with the loss that can come from living with chronic illness. Know that Jesus understands you and that He loves you! This leads me to the next two emotions that I'm going to talk about which are more positive ones!

Hope

"We have this hope as an anchor for the soul, firm and secure." (Hebrews 6: 19) NIV

Hope is something you cannot give up on although there were many times that I did when I was struggling with severe depression. But, as believers, the hope we have is that Jesus died for our sins and that we have a place waiting for us in Heaven where we will live with Him for eternity. What wonderful news! This is the hope I cling to most especially on hard days.

Contentment

"I know what it is to be in need, and I know what it is to have plenty. I have learned the secret of being content in any and every situation, whether well-fed or hungry, whether living in plenty or in want. I can do all this through him who gives me strength." (Philippians 4: 12–13) NIV

Notice that Paul said he learned to be content in his situation. This didn't come easily to him and so we learn that contentment takes time. We can still be content in our situation but hope for better things to come such as healing or a future spouse. For example, you can be content where you are in your health but, still pray for healing. You can be content being single but, still pray for a future husband or wife. You can be accepting of a situation without wanting to stay there. Everything is temporary.

Managing CFS/ME

The importance of self-care

Rest is essential to help manage the symptoms of CFS/ME. Because of this, I have had to be incredibly disciplined when it comes to the nature of rest.

"Love your neighbour as yourself." (Mark 12: 31) NIV

In the church, we are often taught to love and serve others. This of course is great but, you need to love yourself as well! After all, this is what Jesus taught us. So, why do we have such a hard time doing it? One of the reasons I think people struggle in this area so much is because of guilt. I think we can feel guilty if we take time for ourselves or worry about being judged for perhaps being selfish. This is not true! In order to serve others well, you must learn to take care of yourself. I've often heard the phrase, "You cannot serve from an empty teacup," (Chinese scholar Tokusan and Zen Master Ryutan) and this is certainly true!

Here are a few practical tips for rest and self-care:

- Take a nap
- Have a relaxing bubble bath

- Get an early night
- Go for a quiet walk
- Read or listen to some bible verses
- Listen to some calming music
- Have a cup of herbal tea
- Light a candle
- Smell some lavender oil
- Listen to a relaxing meditation

One of the physical triggers for me with CFS/ME is if I catch a virus or a bug, then I'm completely wiped out! This is a sign that I need to increase my rest time.

I am talking as someone who did not know how to take care of myself before. I would run myself into the ground until I had to rest.

"Then, because so many people were coming and going that they did not even have a chance to eat," he said to them, "Come with me by yourselves to a quiet place and get some rest." (Mark 6: 31) NIV

We all have things we need to do – paying the bills, doing the grocery shopping, cleaning the house. I know some of you will have families or spouses and your responsibilities will be different to mine. But, please take time for yourself to rest. It's so important not just to replenish your mind and body but also your soul! This too can be energising.

People pleasing

Am I now trying to win the approval of human beings, or of God? Or am I trying to please people? If I were still trying to please people, I would not be a servant of Christ. (Galatians 1:10) NIV

People pleasing was a big problem for me. I found it hard to say no to people and would often feel guilty if I did say no. I had to learn that God has not called me to be a people pleaser but a God pleaser.

The truth is you can't be all things to all people. Some people aren't going to like everything you do and they're not always going to agree with everything you do. Plus, people-pleasing is exhausting! Living with CFS/ME means I had to start being honest with myself and others about what I can and can't manage. I also had to get good at saying no!

It's okay to say No!

Do you ever feel burdened by all the pressures in life that are coming against you? Rest assured that it is okay to say no to things when you need to.

In the early days of living with CFS/ME, I didn't know how to say no to people. I'd gotten so used to saying yes to everything that I had to start saying no to things. One of the ways I did this was by asking the Holy Spirit to help me.

God would often show me what to do with His peace. If I had peace about doing something, this was often a sign that it was God. On the other hand, if I had a lack of peace about doing something, this was often a sign that it wasn't God! As you go about your days, be aware of God's voice and His leading. Ask Him to show you the next move in everything you do.

"This is what the Lord says – your Redeemer, the Holy One of Israel:

'I am the Lord your God, who teaches you what is best for you,

who directs you in the way you should go.'" (Isaiah 48: 17) NIV

Setting boundaries

It's okay to set boundaries with yourself and others. There's nothing wrong with wanting to protect yourself and keep yourself safe.

For example, try not to approach a potentially stressful situation when your energy levels are low. Or avoid a heated discussion when you're not feeling well. Saying things like, "Can we talk about this another time?" or "I can't manage that right now but maybe later," are good ways of setting boundaries.

We don't always have control over how people treat us but, we do have control over what we allow and how we respond to it. Jesus even encourages us to pray for those who mistreat us and even bless them!

"You have heard that it was said, 'Love your neighbour and 'Hate your enemy'. But I tell you, love your enemies and pray for those who persecute you, that you may be sons of your Father in heaven." (Matthew 5: 43–45) NIV

Practical support

Living with CFS/ME has meant that I've had to be honest about what my limitations are when it comes to the practicalities of life. In the past, I've had cleaners to help me around the house. As I can't make and prepare my own meals, I have meals ready-made for me that I can just microwave in a few minutes. There are a lot of companies now that offer healthy ready-made meals.

Another way of helping me manage is doing my shopping online. This conserves energy and time that I can better spend on other things that I enjoy doing.

Managing your time

As someone who knew how to take a lot on, I had to start managing my time better. That started with how I would plan my weeks and days. Someone once said to me, 'Plan, Pace and Prioritise'. This has stuck with me throughout the years and I now strive to be more balanced in my life.

"Be sober [well balanced and self-disciplined], be alert and cautious at all times. That enemy of yours, the devil, prowls around like a roaring lion [fiercely hungry], seeking someone to devour." (1 Peter 5:8) AMP

One way that has helped me to manage my time better was to pray for wisdom and direction. As I've talked about before, I would often ask God to show me what to say yes to and what to say no to.

Of course, I don't get it right all the time and sometimes I make plans that just don't work out! But, if I can do my part by making some sort of plan in the first place, I can better manage my own time. For example, if I have a busier schedule on one day, I know that I will need to rest more the following day.

Spending time with Jesus

"After he had dismissed them, he went up on a mountainside by himself to pray. Later that night, he was there alone." (Matthew 14: 23) NIV

The most important relationship you will have is with Jesus – our saviour and our closest friend. We all need to nourish and cultivate friendships and relationships in our life but, we need to take time for the best relationship out of them all – Jesus!

Talk to Him about your worries and cares. He longs to hear from you! The more time you spend with Him, the more you will come to know and love Him. He loves you so much!

We see in scripture how Jesus regularly took time away from His ministry to be with the Father. And we need to do the same. This will refresh you and sustain you, especially through hard times.

Doing the things you enjoy!

It's so important to take time for leisure as well as rest. Take time for the things you enjoy in life!

Here are some things you could do:

- o Read a new book
- o Try a new magazine
- o Do something creative like colouring or do a puzzle book
- o Listen to some upbeat music
- o Eat a nourishing meal
- o Meet up with a friend

One of the things I like to do is art therapy. Particularly, on days when my energy levels aren't so good, I might do some mindful colouring or some painting. I also love dancing so, on days when my energy levels are better, I will have a bit of dance! Sometimes I can only manage this sitting down but, it makes me feel better just doing something I love!

Maybe you could do some low-impact energy activities like painting your nails or putting some make-up on? Maybe pamper yourself and try a new face mask?

Also, as I would like to travel one day, I read a travel magazine from time to time. For many years, I was housebound so, I found a gardening magazine quite nice to read so I could look at pictures of nature and pretty flowers. This was quite calming. Also, just sitting by the window and looking out at the beautiful scenery can help improve my mood.

It's also nice to treat yourself! Especially on days when you're not feeling well. Maybe buy yourself some new pyjamas or some chocolate... Chocolate always helps!

Take a break!

Sometimes it's helpful just to take a break from everything. Maybe book a weekend retreat somewhere quiet. I have found this very beneficial in the past when I've needed a change of scene. It's also nice to go somewhere where you can be looked after for a bit!

Another thing you could do is book yourself in for a massage if you can't travel too far. Make time to look after yourself!

Coping with Setbacks

In life, we all go through setbacks which can be very disappointing. We're doing well and life is good then suddenly we hit a setback and quickly become discouraged. During my time living with CFS/ME, there would be times when I was doing pretty well. Then I would go through a relapse maybe from too much activity or catching a virus. This would make me very poorly again and I'd have to go back a few steps. I'd begin to feel very discouraged!

It's okay to feel discouraged but, it's not okay to stay there! We must persevere through these setbacks and not give up on our hopes and dreams.

"Consider it pure joy, my brothers and sisters, [a] whenever you face trials of many kinds, because you know that the testing of your faith produces perseverance. Let perseverance finish its work so that you may be mature and complete, not lacking anything." (James 1: 2–4) NIV

Overcoming weariness

"Do you not know, have you not heard? The Lord God is the everlasting God, the creator of the ends of the earth. He

does not grow weary and His understanding no one can fathom. He gives strength to the weary and increases the power of the weak. Even youths grow tired and weary, and young men stumble and fall, but those who hope in the Lord will renew their strength. They will soar on wings like eagles; they will run and not grow weary, they will walk and not be faint." (Isaiah 40: 28–31) NIV

Living with chronic illness can be hard going! Sometimes we may feel weary from our long suffering but, God has promised to give us strength in such weary times.

One of the things that has helped me manage weariness is leaning on God more, asking Him for more of His presence, peace and comfort. I'm also very open in my relationship with God so I tell Him everything, including how I feel. This can often lead me to take some action to help deal with it. Perhaps, I'll phone a friend or treat myself to something nice.

Sometimes when we feel weary, it's the more practical things we need to attend to such as getting more rest, more sleep or a having good meal. In the Bible, when Elijah was feeling weary, the angel appeared to him telling him he needed to sleep and eat.

"And the angel of the Lord came again the second time, and touched him, and said, Arise and eat; because the journey is too great for thee. And he arose and did eat and drink, and went in the strength of that meat forty days and forty nights unto Horeb the mount of God." (1 Kings 19: 7–8) KJV

Other times, we get weary because we feel the trial has become too much to bear. It's during these times, that we need to remind ourselves of who we are in Christ.

Here are some declarations you can speak over yourself to help combat weariness. When you do this, you are activating your power in the spiritual realms!

I am more than a conqueror through Christ Jesus (Romans 8: 37)

I am an overcomer in Christ (1 John 5: 5)

Nothing is too hard for the Lord (Jeremiah 32: 27)

All things are possible with God (Matthew 19: 26)

Greater is He that is in me than He that is in the world(1 John 4: 4)

I can do all things through Christ who gives me strength(Philippians 4: 13)

I have not been given a spirit of fear but, a spirit of power, love and sound mind (2 Timothy 1: 7) NIV versions

Looking After Your Mental Health

It's just as important to take care of your mental well-being as well as your physical health. I have experience of living with depression and anxiety so, I will talk about what they are and what tools I've found helpful to overcome them.

Depression and anxiety

Depression and anxiety are both serious mental health disorders. I want to make it clear that CFS/ME and depression/anxiety are completely separate health conditions but, one can develop depression/anxiety as a result of suffering with a long-term chronic health condition.

Here's a brief overview of what depression and anxiety are:

What is depression?

Symptoms of depression can include:
Continuous low mood or feelings of sadness
Feelings of hopelessness and helplessness
Low self-esteem

Feelings of guilt or shame
Irritability
Lack of motivation or interest
Difficulty in making decisions
Lack of enjoyment
Loss of appetite
Weight loss or weight gain
More serious symptoms include:
Self-harm
Suicidal thoughts or suicidal attempts

Managing depression

Depression can make you feel really isolated. When I suffered from severe depression, it was like a heavy weight I couldn't move. It was as though I'd lost all hope and given up on myself. As though I couldn't see a way out and nothing ever good was going to happen in my future.

During my times of feeling this way, I would often self-harm and I also had several suicide attempts. It was only when my last serious suicide attempt failed that I realised I needed some help! I needed to be honest with someone about how I was feeling rather than wearing a mask which I was so used to doing. For many years, I would tell people I was doing okay when deep down I really wasn't. Because of this, I struggled in my faith often feeling like God was mad at me and disappointed in me. This just furthered my feelings of guilt and shame which I piled on myself until it was too much to bear.

Sometimes, it's even just too hard to pray when you're struggling with depression and feelings of hopelessness. I want you to know that depression is nothing to be ashamed of. Sometimes, in the church, we can be made to feel like we have to be 'up' all the time! But in reality, this isn't very realistic!

David's story

In the Bible, David was a young Shepherd boy whom God anointed to be King. He was described as *"a man after God's own heart" (1 Samuel 13: 14)* NIV. But many people overlooked him, including his own family.

Throughout, his story we are told of the many successes and failures he experienced in His life. You may know the popular story of David and Goliath. David defeated Goliath a huge Philistine giant who was over nine feet tall with just one stone. At first, Goliath challenged David to a fight thinking he would defeat him.

"Goliath stood and shouted to the ranks of Israel, 'Why do you come out and line up for battle? Am I not a Philistine, and are you not the servants of Saul? Choose a man and have him come down to me. If he is able to fight and kill me, we will become your subjects; but if I overcome him and kill him, you will become our subjects and serve us.'" (1 Samuel 17: 8–9) NIV

However. David was brave enough to volunteer to go and fight Goliath. He had confidence in the Lord that He would deliver and honour him.

"David said to the Philistine, 'You come against me with sword and spear and javelin, but I come against you in the name of the LORD Almighty, the God of the armies of Israel, whom you have defied. This day the LORD will deliver you into my hands, and I'll strike you down and cut off your head.'" (1 Samuel 17: 45–46) NIV

With just one slingshot, David aimed for Goliath's head and killed him.

This is just one of David's success stories but, he also went through many battles. One of them we are told is that he suffered from depression. In Psalm 42: 11, he say*s, "Why are you downcast, O my soul? Why so disturbed within me? Put your hope in God for I will yet praise him, my Saviour and my God."* The Bible with Nicky and Pippa Gumbel, Youth Version, 2024.

David cried out to the Lord in his distress! *"Trust in him at all times, you people; pour out your hearts to him, for God is our refuge." (Psalm 62: 8)* NIV. This is a great lesson to be learnt here that when we are in any kind of distress, we too can cry out to God.

But also notice in Psalm 42: 11 that after David cries out to God, he brings the focus back onto God and he talks about hope!

I'd like to share some scriptures with you that focus on the theme of Hope:

> ➢ *"Therefore, with minds that are alert and fully sober, set your hope on the grace to be brought to you when Jesus Christ is revealed at his coming." (1 Peter 1: 13)*

> *"And the God of all grace, who called you to his eternal glory in Christ, after you have suffered a little while, will himself restore you and make you strong, firm and steadfast." (1 Peter 5: 10)*

> *"And we know that in all things God works for the good of those who love him, who have been called according to his purpose." (Romans 8: 28)*

> *"May the God of hope fill you with all joy and peace as you trust in him, so that you may overflow with hope by the power of the Holy Spirit." (Romans 15: 13)*

> *"There is therefore now no condemnation to them that are in Christ Jesus" (Romans 8: 1)*

> *"I wait for the Lord, my soul waits, and in his word, I hope; my soul waits for the Lord more than watchmen for the morning, more than watchmen for the morning" (Psalm 130: 5–6)* NIV versions

Other practical ways I've found helpful to manage depression are:

> Going for a mindful walk
> Phoning a friend or mental health support worker
> Writing your thoughts and feelings down – it's good to regularly check in with yourself and to be aware of your thoughts and feelings. Rather than bottling them up or keeping them going around in your head, writing them down can be a really helpful way of keeping track of your mood. Maybe then you could talk about them with a trusted friend or someone such

as a professional counsellor or a mental health support worker.

Managing your mood

Learn to laugh!

"A cheerful heart is good medicine, but a crushed spirit dries up the bones." (Proverbs 17: 22) NIV

As the psalmist says, laughter is good medicine! We all go through trials of many kinds but, learning to laugh and maintain a joyful spirit is key to staying strong through them all. *"The joy of the lord is your strength!" (Nehemiah 8: 10)* NIV

Here are some ways you can keep your spirits up!

- o Watch a funny movie or TV show
- o Watch some funny clips online or look at some funny pictures
- o Hang out with a funny friend
- o Laugh at yourself! Sometimes laughing at our own mistakes can take the pressure off. We're all human and we all fall short but, we can see the funny side too.

A thankful heart

"I will give thanks to you, Lord, with all my heart; I will tell of all your wonderful deeds." (Psalm 9: 1) NIV

Making time for gratitude can be a really helpful way of dealing with the frustrations that come along with living with chronic illness and mental health difficulties. Maybe write a list of all the things you can be thankful for today. Even the small things like a warm bed, a comfortable sofa, food in your fridge. These may sound like small things but, in reality, they really are the big things!

What is anxiety?

Being restless all the time

Having a sense of dread or fear that something bad is going to happen

Feeling constantly 'on edge' or hyper-vigilant

Problems concentrating

Feeling irritable

I have suffered from anxiety for a long time but I was only diagnosed when I was in my twenties.

The root of fear

The truth is we live in a spiritual battle. In Ephesians 6: 12, we are told that the battle is not between flesh and blood, *"For our struggle is not against flesh and blood, but against the rulers, against the authorities, against the powers of this dark world and against the spiritual forces of evil in the heavenly realms."* NIV. Therefore, we have a spiritual enemy.

One of the enemy's tactics is to use fear to prevent us from living the peaceful and joyful life that Christ died to give us.

So here are some ways I've found that have helped me manage fear and anxiety.

❖ Prayer and asking for prayer

"Therefore, confess your sins to one another and pray for one another, that you may be healed. The prayer of a righteous person has great power as it is working." (James 5: 16) ESV

This can be a really helpful tool when it comes to managing fear and anxiety as God longs to help us and we cannot do it in our own strength. It's also helpful to open up to people you trust who may be experiencing anxiety too or perhaps some close friends from church that you feel you could ask for prayer from. We need one another and are better together!

❖ Seeking God and His presence

"One thing I ask from the Lord, this only do I seek: that I may dwell in the house of the Lord all the days of my life,
to gaze on the beauty of the Lord and to seek him in his temple." (Psalm 27: 4) ESV

It is a beautiful thing to spend time in God's presence. There we find peace and rest knowing He is sovereign and in complete control. Take time to dwell in His presence and ask Him to fill you with His perfect peace. Spending time in His presence will refresh and renew you!

❖ Worshipping God

"Worship the Lord your God, and his blessing will be on your food and water. I will take away sickness from among you." (Exodus 23: 25) NIV

I have found worship massively helpful in dealing with fear and anxiety. Worship can really help alleviate anxiety as it puts the focus back on God and takes the focus off our worries and cares. Spending time in worship will also refresh and renew your strength.

❖ Listen to the word and Speak it out loud

"Be still and know that I am God." (Psalm 46: 10) NIV

There are many Bible apps available now and online audiobooks that you can listen to in order to help strengthen your faith. Sometimes just having the Bible playing in the background can bring us peace and comfort.

Here are some comforting Bible verses to help you feel more at peace:

"Whoever dwells in the shelter of the Most High will rest in the shadow of the Almighty." (Psalm 91: 1) NIV

"Be still before the LORD and wait patiently for him" (Psalm 37: 7) NIV

"In peace, I will lie down and sleep, for you alone, LORD, make me dwell in safety." (Psalm 4: 8) NIV

"You will keep in perfect peace those whose minds are steadfast because they trust in you." (Isaiah 26: 3) NIV

"God grants sleep to His beloved." (Psalm 127: 2) MEV

"Look to the Lord and His strength, seek His face always." (Psalm 105: 4) NIV

"Cast all your cares onto Him because He cares for you." (1 Peter 5: 7) NIV

Other more practical ways I've found helpful are:

❖ **Writing things down** – sometimes it helps to get things out of our minds. You could journal your anxieties or write things down that you need to do so, it's out of your head and on paper. This may give you some perspective on the problem as well and can help offer a solution. If necessary, you could then talk about it with a friend or someone you trust to get a different perspective on the problem.

❖ **Making plans and having things to look forward to** – Maybe buy a new diary to help plan your days and weeks. It's also good to have things to look forward to so, don't make it all about the to-do's!

❖ **Setting realistic goals** – This can help prevent you from taking too much on and help you be more realistic about what you can manage at the time.

❖ **Get moving!** Sometimes, it can really help just to do something physical (if you can) to distract yourself from your worries. Maybe try a short walk or do some light cleaning around the house just to take your mind off the worry.

❖ **Take it one day at a time** – God's grace is sufficient for the day! You can't live tomorrow's grace today. *"Do not be anxious about tomorrow for tomorrow will be anxious about itself. Each day is sufficient for its own trouble." (Matthew 6: 34)* NIV

If you do find that anxiety or depression are becoming a problem for you, you can always seek professional advice. I take medication for depression and anxiety and there is no shame in that.

Your Worth and Value in Christ

*"Indeed the very hairs on your head are all numbered so do not be afraid; you are worth more than many sparrows."
(Luke 12: 7)* NIV

Living with chronic illness and or mental health can make us feel devalued. We can't do the things everyone else is doing. Maybe we can't go out to work like everyone else or we can't work the number of hours the rest of the world is working. Perhaps you can't go out and visit friends and family. Maybe you feel alone. I want you to know that you are not alone!

It's important to remember that our worth and value are not in what we do but, in who we are as children of God. God is more concerned about who you are in Him and who you are becoming in Him!

Meditate on these truths about what God's word says about you!

- You are God's masterpiece (Ephesians 2: 10)
- You are His Beloved (Ephesians 1: 5–6)
- You are the apple of His eye (Psalm 17: 8)
- You are valuable (Matthew 6: 26)

- You are made in the image of God (Genesis 1: 27)
- You are chosen (Ephesians 1: 4–5) NIV

Appreciate the way God made you and learn to appreciate your value in Him!

Learning to be your own best friend

"You are precious and honoured in my sight and I love you." (Isaiah 43: 4) NIV

Here are some ways you can be a better friend towards yourself:

Encourage yourself!

"David was greatly distressed because the men were talking of stoning him; each one was bitter in spirit because of his sons and daughters. But David found strength in the LORD his God." (1 Samuel 30: 6) NIV

God is for you but are you for yourself? One of the most valuable lessons I have learned is to be my own best friend. Celebrate your progress however small! Maybe you struggle with depression and just getting out of bed was a stepping stone for you today. Or maybe you suffer from a long-term chronic illness and you managed a short walk today.

As I've mentioned before, I've experienced times of loneliness and isolation. During these times, it was especially important that I was my own encourager!

Talk to yourself continually as you would a good friend. You wouldn't be so hard on a good friend of yours so why would you be so hard on yourself? Be your own supporter!

Having self-compassion

"The Lord is gracious and compassionate, slow to anger and rich in love. The Lord is good to all; he has compassion on all he has made." (Psalm 145: 8–9) NIV

Jesus has compassion on you, He understands what you're going through – He knows all too well about suffering. Sometimes, it helps to adopt the same attitude towards ourselves when going through a difficult time. I can be really hard on myself but, sometimes I have to stop and think about all I've gone through and think about what I would say to someone else who has gone through a similar thing. All our stories are unique but, when we all share in the same suffering, we can become stronger together by encouraging and supporting one another through it all. I will talk more about the importance of community later.

Do you like yourself?

"I praise you for I am fearfully and wonderfully made; your works are wonderful I know that full well!" (Psalm 139: 14) NIV

When I was struggling with depression, I really didn't like myself very much! I was very self-critical and would often focus on all my faults rather than what I actually liked about myself. I had to learn to develop a healthy, balanced relationship with myself. The truth is the more you like yourself, the better you're going to get on with other people! Now, I will choose to compliment myself and celebrate my achievements rather than focusing on all my faults and shortcomings.

The Importance of Community

Reaching out to others

"For even as the body is one and yet has many members, and all the members of the body, though they are many, are one body, so also is Christ." (1 Corinthians 12: 12) ESV

Before I got ill, I was a very independent person and I struggled to ask for help. But I have come to learn that I can't do it on my own and I need the help and support of others. We weren't meant to do life alone. We are created for relationships – with God, with ourselves and with others. As I mentioned earlier in the book, there have been times when I've experienced loneliness and there will be times you will experience loneliness too. But God doesn't want us to stay there!

We are called to live in fellowship with one another – community is so important! There were times in my life during years of living with CFS/ME that I was living as though I was an island. I wasn't part of a church although, thankfully I did have support groups online that I could reach out to. But, as I got better and was able to become more involved in a local church, I began to realise the importance of community and reaching out to others.

If you are struggling with CFS/ME and you can't get to church, I would suggest joining some online support groups. There are some great ones that you can join online and it may just help you to have the support and understanding of other people going through the same thing.

I would also encourage you to get involved in a loving, caring church if you can and most importantly, surround yourself with positive, faith-filled people! It's so important who you surround yourself with. If you find the people around you are negative and critical, this can be very draining. You may need to reconsider who you are friends are if you find this to be the case. If you have to put an end to friendships or relationships for this reason, I promise you God will give you new friends!

Asking for help

If you are struggling with CFS/ME, depression, anxiety or any other chronic health condition and are feeling alone, I would strongly advise you to ask for help. Maybe talk to a trusted friend, a professional counsellor or see a doctor. It's okay to admit that you're struggling.

The Waiting Room

"I remain confident of this: I will see the goodness of the Lord in the land of the living. Wait for the Lord; be strong and take heart and wait for the Lord." (Psalm 27: 13–14) NIV

It can be really hard waiting on God. We all have things we're waiting for – healing, a future spouse, and our dreams to come true. Oftentimes, God is preparing us in the waiting period.

This was true for Esther in The Bible. Esther was a beautiful young Jewish woman who was called by God to save her people from annihilation. In the story, King Xerxes is searching for a new queen.

Then the king's personal attendants proposed, "Let a search be made for beautiful young virgins for the king. Let the king appoint commissioners in every province of his realm to bring all these beautiful young women into the harem at the citadel of Susa." (Esther 2: 2–3) NIV

Esther found favour with Hegai who was put in charge of preparing the women to meet the King and she was given special attention. When it was Esther's turn to go before the king, he immediately found her the most attractive and beautiful of all women and placed the royal crown on her head.

"Now the king was attracted to Esther more than to any of the other women, and she won his favour and approval more than any of the other virgins. So he set a royal crown on her head and made her queen instead of Vashti." (Esther 2: 17) NIV

Now, Queen Esther was given a very special assignment by God to deliver the Jews from Haman's plot to kill the Jewish nation. She had to go boldly before the King and request that he save her people. Esther was reluctant at first and she was afraid. Sometimes, when God asks us to do something, we might not want to do it or we might feel afraid.

In order to be ready for what God had called her to do, Esther had to go through a time of preparation so she would be ready to approach the King with her request. One of the ways she had to prepare was by going through times of fasting.

Then Esther sent this reply to Mordecai: "Go, gather together all the Jews who are in Susa, and fast for me. Do not eat or drink for three days, night or day. I and my attendants will fast as you do. When this is done, I will go to the king, even though it is against the law. And if I perish, I perish." (Esther 4: 15–16) NIV

In the same way, sometimes God has to prepare us in order to be ready for what He has in store for us. Queen Esther was afraid but, she took the stand anyway. Sometimes we may feel afraid of doing something hard that God is asking us to do. But, be encouraged! God will give you the grace you need you do it and at the right time, you will be ready.

The story ended well for Queen Esther! Her request was granted by the King and her and Mordecai were honoured with royal garments and a decree was written to protect all Jews.

In the same way, your story can end well too!

Waiting well

Another thing I've learned is the importance of waiting well. There are two ways to wait. Either by getting upset and frustrated because God is not coming through in your time. Or with an expectancy of hope – that better things are to come and with an attitude of patience as we wait for God to come through for us.

I once heard someone say Hope stands for Having Only Positive Expectations. It's a test of trust and the meaning behind it all is to bring us closer to God and trust that the plan He has for us is greater than the plan we have for ourselves and beyond what we could ever imagine!

We don't always understand why God makes us wait. But trust me, when you look back you will!

Have a Dream for Your Life!

"Hope deferred makes the heart sick, but a dream fulfilled is a tree of life." (Proverbs 13: 12) NLT

It's important to have dreams and goals for your life. God gives us dreams and desires for a reason!

In the Bible, Joseph was a dreamer. Joseph was one of the twelve tribes of Israel, the son of Jacob and Jacob's wife Rachel. Known as 'the righteous one', he was highly favoured by his father. His Father even gave him a special, coloured coat. You may know this as Joseph's technicoloured Dreamcoat.

Here's the dream that Joseph was given:

Joseph had a dream, and when he told it to his brothers, they hated him all the more. He said to them, "Listen to this dream I had: We were binding sheaves of grain out in the field when suddenly my sheaf rose and stood upright, while your sheaves gathered around mine and bowed down to it." (Genesis 37: 5–7) NIV

Now, Joseph made the mistake of telling his brothers what the dream was! And as a result, his brothers weren't very happy! They envied him deeply, threw him into a pit and then sold him to buyers in Egypt. Now, as it did for Queen Esther, Joseph's story did end well! He ultimately became ruler of the land, second only to King Pharaoh. But Joesph had to endure many trials on his way to that dream being fulfilled.

When he was sold in Egypt, he was brought by a man named Potiphar who was one of King Pharaoh's ministers. Now, to begin with, it started well! He found success in his master's eye and was appointed head of Potiphar's estate. Things were going well for Joseph!

"The Lord was with Joseph so that he prospered, and he lived in the house of his Egyptian master. When his master saw that the Lord was with him and that the Lord gave him success in everything he did, Joseph found favour in his eyes and became his attendant. Potiphar put him in charge of his household, and he entrusted to his care everything he owned." (Genesis 39: 2–4) NIV

However, Potiphar's wife took a liking to Joseph and tried to seduce him. He was trying to do the right thing and honour God but his actions cost him his title because Potiphar's wife tried to put the blame on Joseph and make out that he was the one who tried to seduce her.

Consequently, Joseph was put in prison where he spent many years abandoned and alone.

"When his master heard the story his wife told him, saying, 'This is how your slave treated me,' he burned with anger. Joseph's master took him and put him in prison, the place where the king's prisoners were confined." (Genesis 39: 19–20) NIV

Already this is a great lesson to be learned that sometimes when you do the right thing and you honour God, the wrong thing happens! But the good news is, even though Joseph spent many years in prison, God was always with him and showed him great favour.

"But while Joseph was there in the prison, the Lord was with him; he showed him kindness and granted him favour in the eyes of the prison warden." (Genesis 39: 20–21) NIV

In the same way, when we go through hardships and trials, God has promised to be with us always. He may not always get us out of the storm but, he will see us through! Also, take note, that when God gives you a dream for your life, it may not happen exactly how you think and it may take longer than you think – as it did for Joseph. But eventually, he made it to second in command to Pharaoh and the dream was fulfilled!

So Pharaoh said to Joseph, "I hereby put you in charge of the whole land of Egypt." Then Pharaoh took his signet ring from his finger and put it on Joseph's finger. He dressed him in robes of fine linen and put a gold chain around his neck. He had him ride in a chariot as his second-in-command and people shouted before him, "Make way!" Thus he put him in charge of the whole land of Egypt. (Genesis 41: 41–43) NIV

God will restore what you lost!

"And I will restore or replace for you the years that the locust has eaten – the hopping locust, the stripping locust, and

the crawling locust, My great army which I sent among you."
(Joel 2: 25)

As we see with Joseph, God not only took him from the pit to the palace but, he restored everything he lost and brought him out better than before! This is a great reminder that what the enemy meant for harm, God will use for good!

"You intended to harm me, but God intended it for good to accomplish what is now being done, the saving of many lives." (Genesis 50: 20) NIV

If you have been struggling with a long-term illness like I have then, be encouraged! God can use it all for good. He can make you a blessing to many. Nothing is wasted with God.

"Instead of shame and dishonour,
you will enjoy a double share of honour.
You will possess a double portion of prosperity in your land,
and everlasting joy will be yours." (Isaiah 61: 7–8) ESV

What a promise to hold onto!

My dream

I have many dreams and desires of my own that I would like to fulfil in my life. Throughout my struggle with CFS/ME and mental health, I have designed a dream board as a way of expressing my hopes and dreams. Even though they have looked far from reach at the time, some of them have actually started to come true! And I'm hoping that the remaining dreams I have will come true as well.

It's great to have a vision for your life and something to look forward to. Start making a list of the things you would like to do in the future. They can be small things such as starting a new hobby or learning a new skill to the bigger things like having a family or having your dream job! Doing this will help keep you encouraged and positive about your future!

What are you passionate about?

"As each has received a gift, use it to serve one another, as good stewards of God's varied grace: whoever speaks, as one who speaks oracles of God; whoever serves, as one who serves by the strength that God supplies – in order that in everything God may be glorified through Jesus Christ. To him belong glory and dominion forever and ever. Amen." (1 Peter 4: 10–11) ESV

One of the ways you can do this is by finding what you're passionate about. God has designed us all uniquely with special gifts of our own. What are yours? What do you love doing?

For example, I am passionate about youth work. I actually wasn't planning on going into youth work but God called me to youth ministry once I graduated from university and I loved it!

I have been able to do bits of volunteering over the years but, I would love to get more involved in this line of work.

"May he grant your heart's desires and make all your plans succeed." (Psalm 20: 4) NLT

If you're not sure what you're gifts are, ask the Holy Spirit to show you the gifts He's given you. Remember, you were put on this earth for a purpose and you have a gift to share with the world that no one else has.

When Life Doesn't Go to Plan!

"Trust in the Lord with all your heart and lean not on your own understanding; in all your ways submit to him, and he will make your paths straight." (Proverbs 3: 5–6) NIV

I can honestly say life has not turned out the way I thought it would. Once I graduated from university, I wanted to pursue a career in media and I wanted to travel the world in my twenties. I didn't expect to get hit with chronic illness and mental health issues at age 21. Nor did I expect it to take so long to get better.

God gave Joseph a big dream for his life, but I'm sure Joseph didn't expect to go through the things he did in order to see his dream come to pass either. As we know, he was mocked by his brothers, thrown in a dungeon, unfairly treated and forgotten about.

Sometimes we feel forgotten or rejected by others too. But God never rejects His people nor, does he ever forget us. *"See, I have engraved you on the palms of my hands." (Isaiah 49: 16)* NIV. We have to hold onto the promise that *'this too shall pass'* when going through difficult times. Hold onto the promises of God and see Him work miracles in your life!

When life doesn't go to plan, it's important to remember that if we knew the plan God has for us, it wouldn't take any faith. Nor would we depend on God for His wisdom and power during the trials of life.

Sometimes life just doesn't go to plan! But we must trust our God through it all because His ways are higher than our ways and His plans are bigger than ours.

"For my thoughts are not your thoughts, neither are your ways my ways," declares the Lord. (Isaiah 55:8) NIV

Sometimes, we fail to see the bigger picture. But, through the twists and turns of it all, we can be assured that God always loves us, He is always for us and nothing can separate us from His love.

"For I am convinced that neither death nor life, neither angels nor demons, neither the present nor the future, nor any powers, neither height nor depth nor anything else in all creation, will be able to separate us from the love of God that is in Christ Jesus our Lord." (Romans 8: 38–39) NIV

Conclusion

Living with CFS/ME and mental health has felt like a 'thorn in the flesh' at times and sometimes it has felt like a burden too heavy to carry. But on the other side, it's sometimes felt like a gift! An opportunity to slow down and re-evaluate what's really important in my life.

I hope you will continue to recover on your own journey with CFS/ME and mental health but, more importantly, I hope it brings you closer to our Heavenly Father and that one day you will get to see Him face-to-face in all His glory!

"For I know the plans I have for you, plans to prosper you and not to harm you, plans to give you hope and a future!" (Jeremiah 29: 11) NIV